FUCK HIIT

Sit down, read, understand and apply.

Your future self will thank you for it.

R&D

Dedications

I dedicate this one to <u>YOU</u> guys.

Without someone willing to read, there is no point in anyone writing

Without someone willing to learn, there is no point in anyone teaching

Without someone willing to apply, there is just no point.

Contents

~~Introduction~~
A wake-up call

HIIT (or High Intensity Interval Training) is ... well, it's just fucking awesome.

Period.

Why the hell wouldn't anyone want to cut their workout time in half, reaping in all the benefits it has to offer whilst leaving you more time to do what's important in your life?? It's a no brainer.

Kind of.

You see, for every shinning glimmer of hope comes the 'I thought it was too good to be true', sneaking up swiftly behind like a creepy old man in an overcoat down a dark alley. But let's be honest, the majority of you reading this (if you haven't already skipped to the workouts section) are looking for the next quick fix and have heard on the grapevine that HIIT will give you all the benefits of that time consuming monotonous exercise you have done in the past, in half the time.

Well, it's true.

What you may not realise, yet though, is that HIIT stands for HIGH INTENSITY interval training. That's right, I said 'high intensity' (in capitals, for effect might I add). If you don't feel like your heart is going to explode out of your chest by the end of your workout, then you my friend, did not train with high intensity.

That's the catch.

In order to reduce your time spent exercising, you MUST replace it with intense, muscle aching, face melting, close to vomit inducing workouts. In other words (and like anything in the world), to get what you want, prepare to work your ass off. This book wasn't written to sell you the idea of HIIT by sugar coating it with chocolate. I'm not Willy Wonka. The idea of it is to be brutally honest with its effectiveness, achieved only through its intensity.

If you choose not to read on after that little statement, I understand and wish you all the best. Sorry you wasted your time, and I hope you find peace and rainbows when you return to 'driving' to the gym to 'walk' on a treadmill (WTF is that all about, really?!) for 60 plus minutes as you read the latest OK magazine telling you how a previously fat celebrity 'tried this one special product and lost 3 stone is a matter of weeks' whilst you simultaneously instagram yourself with a single bead of sweat dripping off your forehead as you plod your way through misery and 'fuck my life' thoughts.

#Helpmebecauseimdyinginside

Back to that celebrity for just a second. Think about this, if any product was that amazing at burning fat or building muscle, it'd be on prescription from the NHS. It'd be damn site cheaper than tummy tucks and ab implants. Has your doctor every recommended 'Belly Buster' pills? I didn't think so.

If you do choose to read on, then congratulations. You've just taken a step forward, and there's hope for you yet.

So why is it so awesome?

Well, it's kind of like the Superman of fitness methods (geek mode – ON) – as in, it can, and will, do everything you need it to in order to make a positive change to your overall health and appearance. It doesn't just make you stronger, like the Hulk, it doesn't just make you faster, like the Flash, or agile like Wolverine – but, with enough time and dedication toward this awesome method of training, you can achieve some amazing things (but no x-ray vision – sorry).

Now I'm not by any means disagreeing with running, biking or any other type of exercise, because they do have their place (and can actually be used as part of HIIT sessions as you'll soon see). What I am saying is that those methods alone are 'missing' that little something for many people. They are boring for most and pretty linear, – running improves your running, cycling improves your cycling, yoga improves your flexibility but HIIT encompasses ALL of that plus more.

What are the benefits of HIIT?

➢ Strips body fat

➢ Targets abdominal fat

➢ Builds lean muscle mass

➢ Improves your VO2 max

➢ Increases bone density

➢ Improves insulin sensitivity

➢ Adds variety to workouts

➢ Requires very little or no equipment

➢ Its time effective

HIIT
(The Sciency bit)

Ok, so you need a little convincing. I don't blame you. I did just write the word 'Sciency' after all. (You just went back to check, didn't you?) Anyway, aside from that, you should know that the fitness industry is full of the latest crazy FAD's and bullshit and I know you're pulling your hair out wondering if this book is as reliable as that last juice diet you went on. You remember the one?! Yeah, that one, where you were promised you would lose 50 pounds of fat in 3 days and wake up on the 3rd day with abs of steel, brand new pearly white teeth, a golden tan and the everlasting energy of a Duracell bunny, and all you had to do was blend and drink a rabbit's foot, 3 frog's eyes and 200ml of unicorn piss. Mmmmm, tasty.

I digress,

The essence of HIIT is very simple:

"Bursts of intense activity followed by periods of less intense activity".

With that in mind, lets break down our benefits so you are sold on HIIT and wonder where it was all your life. Now, I've read books before where the science was so 'out there' I might as well of been reading Klingon. You won't find that here so don't worry. Each heading is broken down into short simple, easy to read nuggets of information.

Strip body fat

The reason why HIIT works so well is because, unlike other conventional methods of fitness, it continues to burn fat up to 48 hours AFTER your workout has ended. Yep. It's true. Burning fat when you aren't working out ... winner. Treadmill crawlers don't get that little benefit.

During High Intensity training, the body has a greater need for oxygen due to the effort you are putting in and thus creates an oxygen shortage, which, in turn, causes your body to ask for more during the recovery phase (after you have finished your workout). This, good people, is known as EPOC or 'excess post oxygen consumption'.

EPOC is the amount of oxygen required to restore your body to its normal resting function, and the human body burns approximately 5 calories for every litre of oxygen you consume.

Bigger oxygen deficit means more oxygen required to obtain equilibrium = more calories burnt.

Target abdominal fat

Now calm down and put your pitch fork away. I assume that you have all heard that you cannot target specific areas of fat, known as 'spot reduction', (if you haven't – I'm sorry to break that you. Also, Santa isn't real and the Earth is not flat). But with HIIT, you have the ability to focus a little more on your abdominal fat than with other methods – so stop doing sit ups – it won't help with losing fat around your midsection!

You gain your fat in areas over your body based largely on your genetics and your hormones. Although there is nothing we can do about your genetics, we can influence our hormones through HIIT whereby we create a metabolic environment that will stimulate the release of a higher than normal amount of abdominal fat compared to steady state exercise such as jogging.

Build lean muscle mass

Let's first get something out of the way for those of you that don't want big muscles because 'eww, that gross'.

Bodybuilders live and breathe lifting weights. They train once or sometimes twice a day, every day – repetitively lifting heavy weights, rep after rep, set after set. They go home and eat their meals to the gram out of their Tupperware, the correct blend of protein, carbs and fats. They get adequate rest to encourage their muscles to recover and grow. They wake up at unsociable hours, just to eat to make sure they don't go into muscle catabolism whilst they sleep. They take an array of supplements daily, some legal, some not legal (careful, we aren't here to judge) to try and get the edge of muscular growth. What I'm trying to say is this:

Even when you want muscles, they are fucking hard to get!

So, a few twenty minute HIIT sessions a week will NOT, by any stretch of the imagination, 100% guaranteed turn you into Arnold Schwarzenegger. So, relax.

When I say build lean muscle mass, I'm taking about an improvement in your 'body composition'. Subtle differences in the way you look. A toned frame that will allow you to carry all that shopping in one trip. To pick up your baby without putting your back out. To change the tyre on your car or even push it off the road. Steady state cardio won't do this as effectively for you as it encourages muscle loss. Picture the body of a 10,000-metre runner compared to that of a sprinter. But, because HIIT is so versatile, if you did want to start looking more muscular, combine it with weight lifting and you have a powerful training programme.

Improve your VO2 max

Your Vo2 max (maximum oxygen consumption) is the maximum rate at which your body can effectively use oxygen during exercise. At some point during training, your oxygen consumption will level out and switch from aerobic (with oxygen) to anaerobic (without oxygen) exercise. Not long after this point, your muscles, fatigued from switching to anaerobic exercise, will force you to stop, due to a build-up of lactic acid.

HIIT will greatly improve VO2 max (meaning you could train at higher intensities for longer periods of time) by forcing your heart and lungs to work harder at short intervals, pumping more oxygen into the muscles, therefore increasing your lactate threshold and your ability to push harder.

Increases bone density

'Bones grow back stronger when you break them'. Have you ever heard that statement? Well, it's true (as long as the break isn't on a joint). Bones grow after experiencing stress. This stress (other than a break, and less painfully) could be from a squat, or a push up, or sprint or any other mechanical overload. Something that is 'weight-bearing'. As stress is applied to the bone, bone cells move to the stressed location and begin laying down new bone to increase the strength in that area. So, running would be great for developing strong bones in the lower body, not so much in the upper body. Swimming, cycling and cross trainers are great for fitness but none of them are weight bearing so don't actually help in creating stronger bones. HIIT on the other hand...

Improves insulin sensitivity

This could be a whole other book entirely, but simply, Insulin sensitivity is how well your body responds to Insulin.

Insulin is a hormone created and released by the pancreas when we take in carbohydrates (and to a lesser extent, protein) which increase blood sugar levels. It acts a key to unlock cells to allow glucose to enter muscles and get used as energy or get stored as fat in order to return blood sugar levels to normal. If you are insulin resistant however, your body has to release more and more insulin to do the same job to reduce the blood sugar levels – thus increasing fat storage. High insulin levels are associated with obesity.

HIIT improves insulin sensitivity because muscles crave glucose during and after exercise. All exercise helps, but HIIT leads the charge because it builds lean tissue throughout the whole body (as we have already discussed) which increases your body's overall demand for energy.

Adds variety to workouts / requires little to no equipment and is time effective

I thought I'd group these altogether as they complement one another. Over the years as a trainer, these are the top 5 reasons I've found of why people stop exercising:

#1. ~~Just Lazy~~. No motivation to change or better themselves

#2. Boredom

#3. ~~You are from the UK.~~ The weather is shit

#4. Gym's are expensive

#5. Donuts are life

Let's focus on numbers 2, 3 and 4. There are always going to be number 1's in the world and number 6 is true. We can't deny it.

So, the other factors of why people quit exercise, the reasons / excuses we can quickly amend are boredom, weather, cost and time.
HIIT will be different every time you train. It won't be run after run after run. Some days you can do a circuit, somedays you can do as many rounds as you can in a set time, some days you can do set exercises every minute on the minute and there are hundreds of exercises out there to scale and change your training session. You will not get bored!
If you live in crappy climates, no problems, you can do HIIT anywhere – including your front room. I reckon Harry Potter could have got an effective HIIT session in and he lived under the stairs! But if one day the weather is way too nice to be indoors – you can take it outside. You don't need a gym for HIIT – but you can use HIIT in a gym if you choose. All you need is what's around you. So HIIT is free, it won't cost

a thing. If you have some equipment at home, great, that can be utilized into your sessions if you so choose.

HIIT sessions can take as little as 6 minutes – who the hell doesn't have 6 minutes in a day to improve their health and wellbeing?

Conclusion

So, there you have it, HIIT is the dog's bollocks and you should start doing it immediately.

It's hard, it pushes you way out of your comfort zone, it'll make you sick and breathless and sweating like a cat trying to bury shit on a marble floor. It'll leave you feeling like you're going to die. Ladies and gents, welcome to real world of working hard to get what you want. There are no magic pills, potions, diets or otherwise that will give you that 'dream body in just 30 days'. It doesn't work that way. The fitness Industry is a mass of companies selling bullshit just to make money, backing it up with photo shopped images of your favorite fitness idols and big bold statements like:

"Fat shredder 2000 will help you lose all of your unwanted bodyfat" *

With tiny little subtext, underneath barely readable like:

*When used in conjunction with a sensible weight loss nutrition and exercise plan

All you need is patience, persistence and perseverance.
You don't own your health, it is borrowed. And your rent is due every day.

So now you know what HIIT is, it's many benefits and why you should do it.

Now I'd like to invite you to take action. Ready??

I almost forgot:

Whenever starting out with an exercise plan, always consult with your doctor to reduce the risk of illness and / or injury.

In short,
"ask your Doctor if getting off your ass is right for you".

Ok. Carry on ....

HIIT workouts

On the following pages, you will find 25 HIIT workouts for you to try out. Beginner or Navy Seal, whatever your fitness level, you will find something challenging.

There are plenty here to get you going and after seeing how HIIT is laid out in the following pages, I'm comfortable you could start tweaking these programs or even writing your own.

It looks so simple yet it works!!

If you've done HIIT before and just wanted some fresh ideas, you're good to go. If you're new to it, just consider the following:

Start with 2 – 3 sessions a week

More is not always better. Intense exercise requires adequate recovery. Especially as a newbie.

Don't do your sessions back to back. Rest at least one day in-between sessions.

Stay hydrated

If you aren't too sure on any of the exercises, may I introduce you to my friends 'Youtube' and 'Google'.

Don't fuck around – just pick a workout and get it done. Train your ass off from start to finish and the results will come.

Enjoy

Legs, Legs, Legs

HIGH KNEES
30 SECONDS
SQUAT JUMPS
20 SECONDS
MARCH IN PLACE
10 SECONDS
REST
30 SECONDS
REPEAT x1

HIGH KNEES
30 SECONDS
MOUNTAIN CLIMBERS
20 SECONDS
MARCH IN PLACE
10 SECONDS
REST
30 SECONDS
REPEAT x1

BURPEES
30 SECONDS
JUMPING LUNGES
20 SECONDS
MARCH IN PLACE
10 SECONDS
REST
30 SECONDS
REPEAT x1

COMPLETE NUMBER OF ROUNDS DEPENDING ON LEVEL OF FINTESS

JUST STARTING OUT - 1 ROUND
DABBLED A LITTLE - 2 ROUNDS
FIT AS FUCK - 3 ROUNDS
SHOW OFF - 4 ROUNDS
BAT SHIT CRAZY - 5+ ROUNDS

The Basics

STAR JUMPS
WALL SIT
PUSH UPS
CRUNCHES
STEP UPS
SQUATS
DIPS
PLANK
HIGH KNEES
LUNGES
PUSH UP ROTATIONS
SIDE PLANK (BOTH SIDES)

COMPLETE EACH EXERCISE FOR 30 SECONDS. REST FOR 10 SECONDS BETWEEN EACH EXERCISE

JUST STARTING OUT - 1 ROUND
DABBLED A LITTLE - 2 ROUNDS
FIT AS FUCK - 3 ROUNDS
SHOW OFF - 4 ROUNDS
BAT SHIT CRAZY - 5+ ROUNDS

Hell on Earth

STAR JUMPS
100
BURPEES
SQUATS
90
BURPEES
BICYCLES
80
BURPEES
SHOULDER TAGS
70
BURPEES
MOUNTAIN CLIMBERS
60
BURPEES
SIT UPS
50
BURPEES
PUSH UPS
40
BURPEES
LEG RAISES
30
BURPEES
JUMPING LUNGES
20
BURPEES
SUPERMANS
10

COMPLETE THE ENTIRE CIRCUIT AS FAST AS YOU CAN. CHOOSE NUMBER OF BURPEES
DEPENDING ON YOUR FITNESS LEVEL

JUST STARTING OUT - 1 BURPEE
DABBLED A LITTLE - 3 BURPEES
FIT AS FUCK - 5 BURPEES
SHOW OFF - 8 BURPEES
BAT SHIT CRAZY - 10 BURPEES

Simple, yet effective

HIGH KNEES
100
SQUATS
10
PUSH UPS
10
V SIT UPS
10

COMPLETE AS MANY ROUNDS OF THE ABOVE CIRCUIT AS YOU CAN FOR TIME

JUST STARTING OUT - 6 MINUTES
DABBLED A LITTLE - 8 MINUTES
FIT AS FUCK - 12 MINUTES
SHOW OFF - 16 MINUTES
BAT SHIT CRAZY - 20 MINUTES

The 'Three'

PULL UPS
5
PUSH UPS
10
SQUATS
15

COMPLETE AS MANY ROUNDS OF THE ABOVE CIRCUIT AS YOU CAN FOR TIME

JUST STARTING OUT - 6 MINUTES
DABBLED A LITTLE - 8 MINUTES
FIT AS FUC K - 12 MINUTES
SHOW OFF - 16 MINUTES
BAT SHIT CRAZY - 20 MINUTES

Jingle 'Bells'

I HANDED KETTLEBELL SWING – LEFT ARM
SQUATS
I HANDED KETTLEBELL SWING – RIGHT ARM
JUMP SQUATS
2 HANDED KETTLEBELL SWINGS
MOUNTAIN CLIMBERS
I ARM KETTLEBELL CLEAN AND PRESS – LEFT ARM
JUMP LUNGES
I ARM KETTLEBELL CLEAN AND PRESS –RIGHT ARM
BURPEES
KETTLEBELL RUSSIAN TWIST
PLANK

IF YOU DON'T HAVE A KETTLEBELL, YOU COULD USE A DUMBBELL

COMPLETE THE ABOVE CIRCUIT FOR TIME PER EXERCISE DEPENDING ON FITNESS LEVEL

JUST STARTING OUT – 20 SECONDS PER EXERCISE
DABBLED A LITTLE – 25 SECONDS PER EXERCISE
FIT AS FUC K – 30 SECONDS PER EXERCISE
SHOW OFF – 45 SECONDS PER EXERCISE
BAT SHIT CRAZY – 60 SECONDS PER EXERCISE

Up Down, Up Down

HIGH KNEES
PUSH UPS
KETTLEBELL SWINGS (OR SQUAT IF YOU DON'T HAVE A KETTLEBELL)
MOUNTAIN CLIMBERS
HIGH KNEES
BICYCLES
DIPS
MOUNTAIN CLIMBERS
HIGH KNEES
BRIDGES

COMPLETE EACH EXERCISE FOR REPS DEPENDING ON FITNESS LEVEL

JUST STARTING OUT – 10 REPS
DABBLED A LITTLE – 15 REPS
FIT AS FUCK – 25 REPS
SHOW OFF – 35 REPS
BAT SHIT CRAZY – 50 REPS

Skipping Hell

SKIP
STAR JUMPS
50
SKIP
JUMPING LUNGES
20
SKIP
TUCK JUMPS
10
SKIP
SQUATS
20
SKIP
HIGH KNEES
60
SKIP
BURPEES
10
SKIP
MOUNTAIN CLIMBERS
40
SKIP
PUSH UPS
20
SKIP
PLANK
60 SECONDS

ALL SKIPPING ROUNDS TO BE 30 SECONDS

COMPLETE ROUNDS OF ABOVE DEPENING ON FITNESS LEVEL. 60 SECONDS REST BETWEEN ROUNDS

JUST STARTING OUT - 1 ROUND
DABBLED A LITTLE - 2 ROUNDS
FIT AS FUCK - 3 ROUNDS
SHOW OFF - 4 ROUNDS
BAT SHIT CRAZY - 5+ ROUNDS

Burn baby, Burn

CIRCUIT 1
STAR JUMPS
20 SECONDS
REST
MOUNTAIN CLIMBERS
20 SECONDS
REST

CIRCUIT 2
JUMPING SQUATS
20 SECONDS
REST
HIGH KNEES
20 SECONDS
REST

CIRCUIT 3
SQUAT JUMPS
20 SECONDS
REST
BURPEES
20 SECONDS
REST

COMPLETE EACH CIRCUIT FOR ROUNDS DEPENDING ON FITNESS LEVEL. THEN MOVE TO NEXT CIRCUIT. ALL REST PERIODS ARE 10 SECONDS

JUST STARTING OUT - 1 ROUND
DABBLED A LITTLE - 2 ROUNDS
FIT AS FUCK - 3 ROUNDS
SHOW OFF - 4 ROUNDS
BAT SHIT CRAZY - 5+ ROUNDS

Son of a Pitch

FULL PITCH SPRINT
WALK BACK TO START TO RECOVER
REPEAT FOR REPS SHOWN BELOW

3/4 PITCH SPRINT
WALK BACK TO START TO RECOVER
REPEAT FOR REPS SHOWN BELOW

HALF PITCH SPRINT
WALK BACK TO START TO RECOVER
REPEAT FOR REPS SHOWN BELOW

PENALTY BOX SPRINT
WALK BACK TO START TO RECOVER
REPEAT FOR REPS SHOWN BELOW

COMPLETE WORKOUT ON SOCCER / FOOTBALL PITCH OR MARK OUT A DISTANCE AT LOCAL PARK

JUST STARTING OUT - 1 SPRINT EACH ROUND
DABBLED A LITTLE – 2-3 SPRINTS EACH ROUND
FIT AS FUCK - 4 SPRINTS EACH ROUND
SHOW OFF -6 SPRINTS EACH ROUND
BAT SHIT CRAZY - 8 SPRINTS EACH ROUND

S'all bout the Speed

SPRINT
SQUAT JUMP
10
JUMP LUNGE
10
REST

SPRINT
SQUAT JUMP
8
JUMP LUNGE
8
REST

SPRINT
SQUAT JUMP
6
JUMP LUNGE
6
REST

SPRINT
SQUAT JUMP
4
JUMP LUNGE
4
REST

COMPLETE AS FAST AS POSSIBLE. REST PERIOD TO BE 30 SECONDS. SPRINT TIMES BELOW

JUST STARTING OUT – 5 SECONDS
DABBLED A LITTLE – 8 SECONDS
FIT AS FUCK – 10 SECONDS
SHOW OFF -15 SECONDS
BAT SHIT CRAZY – 20 SECONDS

Simply Burpees

BURPEES

COMPLETE AS FAST AS POSSIBLE

JUST STARTING OUT – 20 BURPEES
DABBLED A LITTLE – 40 BURPEES
FIT AS FUCK – 60 BURPEES
SHOW OFF - 80 BURPEES
BAT SHIT CRAZY – 100 BURPEES

#Dead

THIS HIIT SESSION REQUIRES THE USE OF A TREADMILL.

GET ON THE TREADMILL BUT <u>DO NOT</u> TURN IT ON.
GRAB THE HANDLES, LEAN FORWARDS AND DRIVE THE BELT WITH YOUR FEET AS FAST AS YOU CAN.
100% ALL OUT-MAX EFFORT!!

SPRINT
JOG IN PLACE
40 SECONDS

COMPLETE FOR 8-12 ROUNDS

JUST STARTING OUT – 5 SECOND SPRINTS
DABBLED A LITTLE – 8 SECOND SPRINTS
FIT AS FUCK – 10 SECONDS SPRINTS
SHOW OFF – 12 SECOND SPRINTS
BAT SHIT CRAZY – 15 SECOND SPRINTS

Double Trouble

STAR JUMPS
KETTLEBELL / DUMBBELL SWING

LUNGES
SQUATS

BEAR CRAWL
PRESS UPS

MOUNTAIN CLIMBERS
BURPEE BROAD JUMPS

BICYCLE
PLANK

COMPLETE EACH PAIR OF EXERCISES FOR 30 SECONDS <u>EACH</u> WITH NO REST. REPEAT FOR
ROUNDS AS SHOWN BELOW THEN MOVE ONTO NEXT PAIR OF EXERCISES

JUST STARTING OUT – 1 ROUND
DABBLED A LITTLE – 2 ROUNDS
FIT AS FUCK – 3 ROUNDS
SHOW OFF - 4 ROUNDS
BAT SHIT CRAZY – 5 ROUNDS

Double Trouble 2

SQUAT TO PRESS (THRUSTERS)
BOX JUMPS

COMPLETE FIRST EXERCISE FOR REPS THEN MOVE IMMEDIATELY ONTO SECOND EXERCISE.
COMPLETE AS FAST AS POSSIBLE

JUST STARTING OUT – 10 REPS EACH EXERCISE
DABBLED A LITTLE – 20 REPS EACH EXERCISE
FIT AS FUCK – 30 REPS EACH EXERCISE
SHOW OFF - 40 REPS EACH EXERCISE
BAT SHIT CRAZY – 50 REPS EACH EXERCISE

Run Forest, run

JUMPING SQUAT
SPRINT
PRESS UP

JUMPING SQUATS AND PRESS UPS ARE DONE FOR 10 REPS EACH.
SPRINT TIME IS SHOWN BELOW.

WHEN COMPLETE, REPEAT FOR 8 REPS EACH, 6 REPS EACH, 4 REPS EACH AND 2 REPS EACH.
SPRINT TIME REAMINS THE SAME THROUGHOUT

JUST STARTING OUT – 5 SECONDS
DABBLED A LITTLE – 8 SECONDS
FIT AS FUCK – 10 SECONDS
SHOW OFF -15 SECONDS
BAT SHIT CRAZY – 20 SECONDS

Travelling in Style

SET UP 2 CONES 10 METRES APART

STARTING AT ONE CONE, COMPLETE THE FOLLOWING EXERCISES, TRAVELLING BETWEEN THE TWO CONES.
WALK BACK TO THE START AT AND REPEAT FOR ROUNDS SHOWN BELOW

JOG
SPRINT
CRAB WALK
2 FOOTED JUMPS
BEAR CRAWL
LUNGE WALK
BURPEE BROAD JUMP

JUST STARTING OUT – 1 ROUND
DABBLED A LITTLE – 2 ROUNDS
FIT AS FUCK – 4 ROUNDS
SHOW OFF -6 ROUNDS
BAT SHIT CRAZY – 8 ROUNDS

Sk-urpees

SKIP
50 PASSES
BURPEE
1
SKIP
40 PASSES
BURPEE
2
SKIP
30 PASSES
BURPEE
3
SKIP
20 PASSES
BURPEE
4
SKIP
10 PASSES
BURPEE
5

COMPLETE AS FAST AS POSSIBLE FOR ROUNDS DEPENDING ON FITNESS LEVEL

JUST STARTING OUT – 1 ROUND
DABBLED A LITTLE – 2 ROUNDS
FIT AS FUCK – 3 ROUNDS
SHOW OFF -4 ROUNDS
BAT SHIT CRAZY – 5 ROUNDS

Repetitive Strain

BURPEES
3
V SIT UPS
5
PUSH UPS
5

COMPLETE ALL 3 EXERCISES BACK TO BACK EVERY MINUTE ON THE MINUTE FOR TIME. DEPENDING ON FITNESS LEVEL. THE QUICKER YOU COMPLETE THE 3 EXERCISES, THE MORE REST YOU GET.

JUST STARTING OUT – 4 MINUTES
DABBLED A LITTLE – 6 MINUTES
FIT AS FUCK – 10 MINUTES
SHOW OFF -14 MINUTES
BAT SHIT CRAZY – 20 MINUTES

Repetitive Strain 2

SKIP
25 PASSES
JUMPING SQUATS
5
PUSH UPS
5

COMPLETE ALL 3 EXERCISES BACK TO BACK THEN REPEAT CONTINUALLY FOR TIME. REST ONLY WHEN YOU NEED TO

JUST STARTING OUT – 6 MINUTES
DABBLED A LITTLE – 8 MINUTES
FIT AS FUCK – 12 MINUTES
SHOW OFF -15 MINUTES
BAT SHIT CRAZY – 20 MINUTES

Standard

SQUATS
5
PUSH UPS
5
SIT UPS
5

COMPLETE ALL 3 EXERCISES BACK TO BACK THEN REPEAT CONTINUALLY FOR TIME. REST
ONLY WHEN YOU NEED TO

JUST STARTING OUT – 5 MINUTES
DABBLED A LITTLE – 8 MINUTES
FIT AS FUCK – 12 MINUTES
SHOW OFF -15 MINUTES
BAT SHIT CRAZY – 20 MINUTES

300

PULL UPS
PUSH UPS
SQUATS

COMPLETE ALL 3 EXERCISES FOR REPS SHOWN BELOW, AS FAST AS POSSIBLE

JUST STARTING OUT – 15 REPS PER EXERCISE
DABBLED A LITTLE – 30 REPS PER EXERCISE
FIT AS FUCK – 50 REPS PER EXERCISE
SHOW OFF -75 REPS PER EXERCISE
BAT SHIT CRAZY – 100 REPS PER EXERCISE

32 Rounds of Joy

PULL UPS
8 ROUNDS
PUSH UPS
8 ROUNDS
SIT UPS
8 ROUNDS
SQUATS
8 ROUNDS

COMPLETE EACH EXERCISE FOR TIME SHOWN BELOW. REST AND THEN REPEAT. 8 ROUNDS
TOTAL. THEN MOVE TO NEXT EXERCISE

JUST STARTING OUT – 10 WORK / 15 REST
DABBLED A LITTLE – 10 WORK / 10 REST
FIT AS FUCK – 15 WORK / 15 REST
SHOW OFF -15 WORK / 10 REST
BAT SHIT CRAZY – 20 WORK / 10 REST

10/15/20

PUSH UPS
10
V SIT UPS
10
SUMO SQUATS
10
PUSH UPS
15
V SIT UPS
15
SUMO SQUATS
15
PUSH UPS
20
V SIT UPS
20
SUMO SQUATS
20
REST
1 MINUTE

COMPLETE ENTIRE CIRCUIT AS FAST AS POSSIBLE THEN REPEAT FOR ROUNDS DEPENDING ON FITNESS LEVEL

JUST STARTING OUT – 1 ROUND
DABBLED A LITTLE – 2 ROUNDS
FIT AS FUCK – 3 ROUNDS
SHOW OFF -4 ROUNDS
BAT SHIT CRAZY – 5 ROUNDS

Gamechanger

BURPEES
SQUATS
SIT UPS

REST
1 MINUTE

ALL 3 EXERCISES BACK TO BACK = 1 RD (ROUND)
COMPLETE 5 ROUNDS BASED ON REPS SHOWN BELOW

JUST STARTING OUT – RD 1-10/RD 2-10/RD 3-10/RD 4-10/RD 5-10
DABBLED A LITTLE – RD 1-20/RD 2-10/RD 3-10/RD 4-10/RD 5-10
FIT AS FUCK – RD 1-30/RD 2-20/RD 3-10/RD 4-10/RD 5-10
SHOW OFF - RD 1-40/RD 2-30/RD 3-20/RD 4-10/RD 5-10
BAT SHIT CRAZY – RD 1-50/RD 2-40/RD 3-30/RD 4-20/RD 5-10

Ta Daaa

And that is that.

Thanks so much for taking time out and choosing this book, I hope it helped in some way.

I'd love to get your feedback on this book and use it to make any changes / updates in the future to give yourselves and other readers a better reading experience. If you think it's absolutely amazing and has helped you in some way, I'd love to read about that too (who wouldn't?!), so please feel free to leave a quick review on Amazon to help other people who are / were in the same boat as you and are looking for inspiration and help to make that change.

Please feel free to check out my other books on Amazon:

Fuck burpees

20 ways to influence muscle growth (no drugs required)

Printed in Great Britain
by Amazon